Flat Belly Tea Diet

Lose 10lbs of Fat in a Week with this Revolutionary New Plan

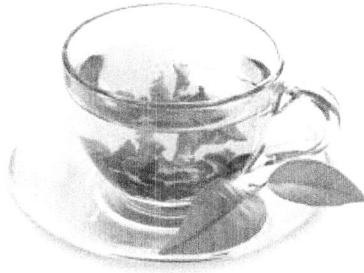

Melinda Rolf

Table of Contents

Introduction

A flabby tummy is never a good thing.

You might lose confidence; feel like you can't do anything and your energy levels will suffer too.

In short, it's something that you probably don't want to deal with.

But, with the help of this book, you'll learn how to let go of that flabby tummy, and replace it with a flat tummy in just 2 weeks or a little more—through the help of the Flat Belly Tea Diet

By reading this book, you will know which kinds of tea to drink, how tea helps you lose weight, how to be a tea ceremony master, and, you'll also be treated to various recipes that you can make to add tea in your diet—All of which will help you reach your ideal weight in no time!

What are you waiting for?

Read this book now and find out how!

How Does it Work?

One amazing thing about tea is that it rids the body of toxins, which makes it such a powerful drink. You've probably heard about detox diets, but may not have thought about tea as a main component of the diet.

Well, you can now tell yourself that it's always beneficial to keep tea at home—because you can use it for cleansing, and for removing toxins away from your body. Here are some basic tips as to how you can use tea for detox.

Refresh

The first part of the Flat Belly Tea Diet is called *Refresh*, and it also consists of two parts, mainly refresh in the morning, and cleansing at night.

What you have to keep in mind is that refresh is all about replacing lost electrolytes and vitamins that may have left the body after cleansing. If you by-pass this step, the detox will not work the way it's supposed to—and that's not what you want to happen at all.

So, what should a refresh tea be like?

Well, for starters, you have to remember that it should be filled with vitamins and anti-oxidants. It's said that Matcha (Green Tea) is a good tea to start with, and you can add the following ingredients.

Spirulina –freshwater type of algae that regulates blood sugar levels, and lessens the amount of cholesterol in the body, due to its high protein content.

Barley Grass – Barley is considered a major cereal grain, which makes it an amazing source of fiber.

Ginseng – Ginseng lowers blood sugar levels and generally boosts the immune system.

Acai Berry – Acai berry is the fruit of the Acai palm tree, and contains an incredible amount of antioxidants that refreshes the body thoroughly.

Just take note, though, that the taste might be strange, you may not like it at first but over time you will become accustomed to it. So stick with it.

Cleaning the Colon

Colon cleanse is another important aspect of the diet, which is of course, about ridding the colon of toxins that make the body weak and susceptible to diseases. The main ingredient you should use is something called Senna Leaf.

Senna Leaf is mainly used as a laxative, which prevents irritable bowel syndrome, and constipation. It's also essential in helping one lose weight, as well as in the treatment of hemorrhoids.

The leaf has quite a strong taste, but you can expect the fruit to be gentler.

Now, all you have to do is make sure you're able to create a great and soothing blend that will help you feel better—and make the act of cleansing your colon easy. You can do that by adding the following:

Licorice Root – Licorice prevents stomach inflammation, and keeps the colon free from toxins. It's also great in the prevention of stomach ulcers, colic, and heartburn, and is also used to treat cough, bronchitis, and sore throat. It's been said that Licorice Root may prevent food poisoning.

Lemon Grass – Lemon Grass is mainly used in the treatment of digestive spasms, as well as achy joints, cough, pain, convulsions, and high blood pressure. It's also used in the prevention of muscle pain, and aromatherapy.

Nettle Leaf – If you're experiencing urinary tract problems, you can always count on nettle leaf to help you out. It's also used as an astringent, a diuretic, and can prevent and treat ailments of the joints, and alopecia (hair loss).

Dandelion – Dandelion has amazing anti-bacterial properties and can also help heal wounds fast. Dandelion is also used in the prevention and treatment of gall stones, kidney stones, and heart weakness. It's also a powerful tonic.

Dried Orange Peel – the scent and taste of orange peel is great in soothing the body, and because orange is a citrus fruit, it keeps you protected from various diseases, too.

The Schedule

Of course, keeping a proper tea detox schedule is important. Here's what you should keep in mind:

It all starts with what you'll do in the morning. Basically, what you should do is boil water, and then add ginger and lemon juice or lemon slices in the mix. This way, your metabolism will be kicked up because you are giving your organs a "wake up call"

After 20 minutes, it's time to make your refresh tea. Take a cue from what was said earlier—this tea will give you an energy boost that will last throughout the day.

Of course, you also shouldn't go through your day without drinking other kinds of tea. It's always best to drink green tea, whether normal blend, or with added ingredients, such as jasmine. White tea might be good, too. Try to take 3 to 6 cups of tea throughout the day.

Night time is always meant for a colon cleanse. Make tea based on the ingredients that were mentioned earlier.

Make sure that you follow the schedule for 1 to 3 weeks at a time, and take note that it's also important to change meal plans from time to time, just like in any other kind of detox diet.

The Tea Ceremony and How to become a Tea Ceremony Master

One of the things that can help you understand the importance of tea better is the Japanese tea ceremony, also more simply known as the tea ceremony. In this chapter, you will know everything you need to learn about it!

What Is the Tea Ceremony?

Originally known as a Japanese artistic pastime, the tea ceremony is about serving and drinking *Matcha* (Japanese green tea).

In the 14th century, members of the upper class started to make Matcha a big part of their social gatherings, as a means of appreciating Chinese crafts and paintings while in a peaceful atmosphere, mostly in a *Shoin*, or study room.

You see, Matcha didn't really originate from Japan, but from China. Matcha arrived in Japan in the 8th century, and started being popular around the 12th century. In Japan, the process of serving and drinking tea is considered a spiritual practice—that's why they have great respect for those who know how to do the tea ceremony well.

Why Does it Happen?

Basically, the tea ceremony is performed to foster a friendly and relaxed atmosphere between the host and his guest. It heavily relies on *Temae,* also known as the etiquette of serving tea that has connections to Zen Buddhism, calligraphy, ceramics, art, and flower arrangement, among others—more on this later.

The Way of the Tea

The Tea Ceremony is also known as *Sado* or *Chado*, which literally means the way of the tea, which doesn't only talk about the ceremony itself, but the process of learning and devoting time to mastering the ceremony.

The Way of the Tea is based on the tea philosophy, which covers:

> **Kei/Respect.** According to the ceremony, it's important that people respect everything around them, and should not think that just because they're humans it means that they're above everyone else. To understand that everyone is their equal, they have to pass through a small entrance (also called *Nijiriguchi*) for them to be allowed entry to the room. Then, they will kneel and bow down to the scroll, and sit beside one another at the tatami mat. Careful handling of the tea bowl and other objects in the room is also considered a sign of respect.

Wa/Harmony. The element of harmony in nature should be present in the room, which means that utensils have to complement each other, and that colors have to be in one theme, too. Also, you have to keep in mind that the tea garden has to reflect the flowers and plants surrounding it.

Sei/Purity. Once inside the room, the person has to let go of his worries and thoughts, so that once the ceremony starts, he can just enjoy what's going on around him, and he can refresh and revitalize him/herself, too. The cleaning of utensils signifies purity, as well. The ceremony also should be done from the heart, and not just through memorization.

Jaku/Tranquility. Once respect, harmony, and purity are achieved, tranquility can finally happen.

Wabi/Appreciation. Next comes the appreciation of all natural things, as well as understanding that nature's beauty is different from what society dictates. Take note that the room's interiors do not have to be perfect. Untreated and unpainted beams and pillars are okay.

Kokoroire/Pouring of Tea. And finally, Kokoroire, or pouring your heart into tea, which will then complete the whole ritual of *The Way of the Tea.*

The Design of the Garden
This will serve as a guide as to how the garden should look like for the ceremony.

The Waiting Area/ Kosikake-Machiai. From the shelter, (this is where the guests will stay while waiting for the host of the ceremony). Usually, this area is filled with woven rush, and an ashtray on the side. Heaters are also important during colder months so guests can warm their hands.

Garden Path/ Roji. One thing that you have to keep in mind when it comes to designing the garden path is that it has to give guests the feeling that they're now entering a different world. It has to be filled with stepping stones, 60% of which will be for walking, while 40% will be for decorative purposes. Make sure that those stones are easy to walk on. Colored stones should then be used as decorations for this path.

The Purifying Basin/Tsukubai. This is where the guests are supposed to pour water over their hands. They will also be drinking from the palm of their hands as a form of cleansing the body and the soul. This should be made from stone, with water dripping from the bamboo pipe. You can take a look at Japanese temples and gardens, for inspiration.

Utensils Used

Here is a list of the utensils that you have to prepare for this occasion:

Hemp Cloth/Chakin. This is a rectangular white hemp or linen cloth that's used to clean the tea bowl after guests are done drinking. After washing the cloth, it has to be stretched out so there are no creases around, and it also has to be folded in a 2/3 manner (2 times-length; 1/3 width). It is placed on the lit kettle during the ceremony itself.

Tea Caddy/ Cha-ire. The tea caddy usually has a gold leaf on its underside and must also have a lid made from ivory. The whole caddy itself has to be made from ceramic materials. Cha-ire is used for thick tea and has to be cleaned first before being used to scoop green tea. Once guests are finished drinking, they could then take turns in viewing the tea caddy

Tea Whisk/ Chasen. A single piece of bamboo is used to create the tea whisk for the ceremony. Bamboo may either be fresh, dried, or smoked, and you can also decide whether their heads have to be fine, rough, or medium. The type of tea whisk used will always depend on the kind of tea being served.

Tea Bowl/ Chawan. This is considered as the most important element of the ceremony, particularly because this is what guests will be drinking from. Without the tea bowl, the tea wouldn't even get to be served! Deep bowls are used during winter to keep tea warm for a long time, while shallow bowls are used during summer. Bowls can also be named by their creators, or even tea masters who use them most of the time. It's also okay if they're imperfect or irregular, because their imperfections only make them seem more real. However, if a tea bowl is really broken, it can be repaired with the help of powdered gold—which then disguises its color, and powdered gold can also be used to create more designs in the future.

Silk Cloth/Fukusa. There's also a silk cloth, otherwise known as Fukusa, that's used for ritual cleansing purposes, as well, and is usually monochromatic and unpatterned; but there are a few instances when patterned ones are okay. Women have to use those in colors of red and orange, while men have to use purple cloth. The cloth is also used by guests to protect implements of the tea, too.

Hemp Cloth/Fukin. Fukin is the term given to another piece of hemp cloth that's used to wipe the bowl after green tea has been served. It's also used to prevent tea spillage.

Kettle-Lit/Futa. This is the term given to the kettle's lit, and is usually shaped differently, and is made from iron.

Portable Brazier/Furo. During the summer and spring seasons, Furo, a Portable Blazer, is used. It's made from clay or iron. It is then placed on a lacquered board so burning can be prevented. There should also be a cut opening, which will serve as a fire window, and a bed of ashes will then be laid inside the Furo. The range used for this must be smaller than other fire ranges

Ladle/Hishaku. The ladle is made from a long piece of bamboo, and has a nodule on its handle. This is mainly used to get hot water from the pot to the bowl, and is sometimes used to handle fresh water. It is also sometimes displayed before the start of the ceremony. The size of the ladle varies, depending on the occasion.

Lit and Ladle Rest/Futa Oki. To keep Furo warm, Futa Oki should be kept in its place, and the bamboo ladle must then be placed inside. You should then hold the ladle in your left hand, and have this help you get the first scoop of warm water for the tea. The ladle must then be placed inside when it's not being used.

Fire Bowl/Hibachi. The fire bowl is used during preparation only. This may either be a wooden box or a large earthen pot.

Kettle or Iron Pot/ Kama or Chanoyugama. Meanwhile, the kettle or iron pot is used to heat water for the tea. Their mouths may take on various shapes, and do not have to be symmetrical at all.

Cold Water Container/Misuzashi. As the name suggests, it's mainly used to store cold water.

Waste Water Bowl/ Kensui. After the ceremony, water has to be poured into waste water bowls to prevent trash from accumulating in the room. It should be cylindrically-shaped, and made from either metal or clay. Don't ever reuse water in front of guests as it's considered to be offensive and rude.

Drawstring Pouch/Shifuku. The tea caddy is usually placed inside a drawstring pouch first that's made from striped silk, damask, and high quality silk brocade. The drawstring pouch is also considered as one of the most valuable items in the ceremony.

Sunken Hearth/Ro. Meanwhile, the sunken hearth is usually used during fall or winter—or anytime the weather is cold. A hole is created on the tatami mat so the sunken hearth can have a place to stay in. Seeing it also provides guests with the feeling that the place is warm and inviting.

Water Pitcher/ Yakan. And finally, you have the water pitcher, also known as Yakan, which is used to refill the cold water container at the end of the ceremony. It is said that this brings the ceremony to an end, in the sense that the room is brought back to its original state.

Preparing for the Ceremony

Preparing for the ceremony is done in two ways, one for the summer, and another for the winter season. Here's how it is done.

Furo Preparation (Summer Preparation)

During summer, here's what should happen:

First, don't forget to send invitations to your guests.

Clean the garden and get the utensils to use for the ceremony

Proceed to prepare the tearoom, and don't forget to clean the sliding doors, and the Shoji paper there.

Next, make sure to replace the tatami mats.

Prepare the meal—you can do this even on the day before, or on the morning before the ceremony.

Make sure that you're ready for any emergencies or unforeseen events that may happen.

Before opening the door, take note that you have to place the Higashi sweets on the tatami mat.

Now, when you open the door of the tea room, make sure that you do so with both hands—as this is considered a warm welcoming gesture. In case the door slides to the left, it has to be opened yet again. Use your right hand and make sure it crosses in front of your body.

Once the door is open, it's time to present the sweets to the guests. You will then stand up in a smooth movement, and use your left foot first in moving towards the guests, and then sit down and place the bowl next to them. You will utter the words *Okashi Wo Dozoo*, which literally means *please, have these sweets*. Do so while bowing to the guests. They should also bow in a silent manner.

Next, you must go and bring the utensils. Start with the cold water container, followed by the portable blazier; after which, the tea bowl should be brought in, carried in the left hand. It must be placed directly in front of the cold water container. Hemp cloth and tea whisk have to be brought in next, followed by lit rest, ladle, and kettle lit.

Greet the guests once again with a bow, and guests must then follow suit. Arrange the clothes used for the ceremony, and then go ahead and sit—just make sure that everyone's comfortable, though. Take a deep breath so you can all go into a meditative state—to contribute to the serenity of the room. Then, prepare the best bowl of green tea that you can make, and then move it close to your knees lightly.

The tea bowl is then picked up using the right hand, and brought down using the right hand, as well. The hemp cloth should then be folded using the left hand, and the bowl must be wiped with it.

The lit is then removed using the left hand, and placed next to the ladle rest using the right hand. Scoop water right out of the pitcher into the bowl, using the right hand's index and middle finger to lift it up. Serve the tea using the left hand, aided by the right hand, so that the guests are facing forward upon receiving the tea.

After serving and clearing waste water, you can go and make tea again, provided that all of you are up for some more tea.

Ro Preparation (Winter Preparation)
Preparing for a winter ceremony is very similar to how it is done during summer, but you have to remember two important things, which are:

Men should always sit diagonally from the center of the table, with the cold water container on their side. They must place the ladle and bowl next to the brazier. The cold water container is then turned in a counter-clockwise motion, and has to be placed parallel to one's legs. After doing so, the host should greet the guests and tell them that he will already start making tea. The host must also adjust the clothing and relax his breath. Also, make sure everyone's comfortable in their sitting positions as they will stay that way for the rest of the ceremony.

Women, meanwhile, should sit straight and face the cold water container each time they put a utensil down. The ladle cover should be placed at least 3 centimeters away from the blazier, and holding utensils must be done in an angle that is perpendicular to the left side of the chest. The ladle rest should be held at stomach height and moved in clockwise motion at all times. The host must greet the woman and tell her that he is about to start making tea specifically for them. Cloth adjustment should be done during this time, too. You should do so by saying *Ippuku Wo Sashiagemasu*.

Types of Tea Ceremony

There are also various kinds of ceremony that are based on the times of the day that they're being done. These are:

First Use of the Portable Blazier of the Year / Shoburo. Basically, this ceremony is done to celebrate the arrival of the year's first blazier.

Winter Dawn Ceremony/ Akatsuki No Chaji. As the name suggests, this ceremony is held early in the morning (i.e., at dawn) so that guests can enjoy the breaking of the dawn while in the tearoom.

Winter Early Evening Tea Ceremony/ Yuuzari-No-Chaji. This is the ceremony that is meant to allow guests to appreciate the experience of being in daylight, up to sunset. It is said to bring a mystical feeling to the guests.

Summer Early Morning Tea Ceremony/ Asa-Cha. This is usually done during a hot summer morning, but it can be quite tricky because you have to make sure that the coal isn't that hot—so it won't make the guests uncomfortable.

Breaking New Tea Jar Seal/ Kuchikiri-No-Chaji. Usually, Japanese get new tea jars on the 7th or 8th of November, and they celebrate it with a tea ceremony, of course. The tea jar may not really be directly bought from the store, but may be something that has been sitting in the house for a while. The ceremony should only happen once the tatami mats have been changed, and when seals of the new jars have been broken—to signify new beginnings.

Ceremony Honoring the Last Amounts of Tea/ Nagori-No-Chaji. Well, as the name suggests, the ceremony is all about celebrating the fact that there is still some tea left in the jar. This usually happens during the last few weeks of October.

Winter Evening Tea Ceremony/ Yobanashi. This ceremony is meant to celebrate long winter nights (Winter Solstice). During this ceremony, the tea room and garden may also be decorated with lanterns and lights of different kinds.

Boiling of the First Kettle Ceremony/ Hatsugama. If you attend a tea school, you will learn that this is a special tea ceremony because the tea master/teacher will be the one who will make the tea himself—and will serve it to his students, too!

How to Be a Tea Ceremony Master

To be a master of the tea ceremony, you can either go to a tea school (Yes, they have tea schools in Japan) or read books that will help you develop your tea-making skills. As they say, it is best to witness the ceremony with your very own eyes. Some museums may have a tea ceremony so check them out. Let's start with the schools first..

Urasenke. Urasenke is said to be the tea school with the biggest following. It is known for facing the back street, and has been around since the 1600s. It's also known as the *House of the Sen.*

Mushanoukoujisenke. This tea school was established by the grandson of Urasenke's creator. It's a tea school that faces both streets.

Omotesenke. The school is popular for using smoked bamboo for its tea bowl. It's also said to be the best school that teaches students how to properly arrange utensils and the like.

It may also help if your read these books for reference:

1. Japanese Tea Ceremony – Seno Tanaka
2. Chado: The Way of the Tea – Sasaki Sanmi
3. Cha-No-Yu: Japanese Tea Ceremony - A.L. Sadler
4. The Book of Tea – Kakuzo Okakura
5. Tea Life, Tea Mind – Soshitsu Sen
6. The Japanese Way of Tea – Sen XV Shositsu
7. Rediscovering Rikyu – Herbert Plutschow
8. Tea and Buddhism – Ryofu Pussel

And of course, remember: Practice always makes perfect!

How Tea Can Help You Lose 10 lbs. in a Week

Since we're talking about detox and cleansing, you probably already have an idea that it will help you lose weight, too.

But, how exactly does tea work to help you lose weight? Here's what you need to know.

Tea Metabolizes Fat

Especially green tea. This happens when tea is broken down in the digestive tract—so it can then make its way through the bloodstream. What happens is that fat burning hormones are activated with the help of the compounds present in green tea. This is mainly due to EGCG, tea's most abundant catechin.

What is EGCG?

EGCG, also known as Epigalocatechin Gallate, is a polyphenol that has the same effect as most dietary supplements, which is used to boost metabolism. Research also has it that EGCG can be used to prevent cancer, and maybe even HIV—but studies are still being done to prove the latter.

EGCG is also important because it aids in breaking down *Norepinepherine*, a neurotransmitter that's essential in cognitive alertness. It helps make someone more attentive, and also builds empathy, so the person could relate to others better. It improves one's flight-or-fight response, as well.

Now, Norepinepherine tells fat cells to break the amount of fat in the body down, and release the broken fat into the bloodstream so it can then be turned into ketones that help make a person more energetic, and adept in doing what he has to do.

Tea Has a Few More Substances That Help You Lose Fat

Aside from EGCG, tea contains other elements that aid in weight loss.

Among these is caffeine, which is also an essential part of coffee, and has a lot of potent biological effects. Tea has less caffeine than coffee or soda, though, and that's why those who drink it don't really get annoying side-effects, such as palpitations, headaches, and the like.

Of course, Caffeine helps one lose weight as it is known as a stimulant. It works two ways, which are:

It burns calories. Caffeine particularly stimulates thermogenesis, which is the way the body uses heat to generate energy through the help of various food sources.

It suppresses the appetite. Caffeine reduces one's desire to eat for a certain amount of time.

Make sure, though that you only take caffeine from tea, because drinking tea and coffee simultaneously might just create undesirable side effects; but since tea contains less than 400 milligrams of caffeine (the acceptable amount), you should be just fine..

And of course, there are also catechins (an example is EGCG) that oxidize hormones in order for them to tell fat cells to break themselves down, and turn themselves into energy. Catechins also reduce the amounts of fat inhibitors in the body, which you can benefit from whether by drinking tea, or taking tea extracts.

Tea Is a Good Exercise Aid

Since tea promotes fat burning, you can expect that when taken after exercising, it'll significantly boost the effects of the said exercise, especially when taken in a matter of 8 weeks, and you can expect the effects to stay in the long run.

Tea Automatically Helps You Take in Fewer Calories

As mentioned earlier, tea contains caffeine that suppresses appetite, which means that your body will take fewer calories than usual. More so, research has it that tea can reduce the amount of fat that people get from other food sources. Basically, you can keep in mind that tea burns fat, which in turn, helps your body realize that it doesn't have to take a lot of calories in.

Tea Drives Dangerous Fat Away

At the same time, tea also drives the dangerous fat away from the body, so all you can take in is healthy abdominal fat—which of course, will not make you fat. This way, you can be sure that the kind of fat that's in your body is the one that can help organs function the way they're supposed to, as opposed to breaking them down. This means that with the right amount of fat and calories, you will be able to protect yourself from various diseases.

Things to Remember

You have to keep in mind that tea will not only by itself. Make sure that you add a lot of protein and carbohydrates in your diet, too. You can start with the following:

Lean chicken, fish, veal, lean beef, non-fat mozzarella cheese, chicken breast, pork loin, watermelon seeds, squash seeds, pumpkin seeds, nuts, eggs, mature soy beans, French beans, Lima Beans, tofu, soymilk, milk, and yogurt.

Also, make sure to keep the following in mind:

Chew your food slowly. You know, most fast eaters end up with bloated bellies because they don't take time to chew their food. The thing with not chewing food slowly is that you end up sucking too much air which can lead to bloating. So, take your time when eating. Remember, eating isn't a race—make sure that you enjoy your food, and that you eat properly.

Stay away from chewing gum. Chewing gum also makes you suck in more air than necessary. Sometimes, it's hard to stay away from chewing gum, though, because it may have become a habit. What you can do is just choose other healthy food when you're in need of a good snack. Try low-fat popcorn, fruits, and vegetables instead.

Don't drink carbonated drinks too much. Carbonated drinks (even low-cal/diet ones) just trap gas inside your body, so if you're not a big fan of water, you can spruce it up a bit by adding lime, lemon, or orange—to turn it into flavored water. Peppermint tea may help as well.(See recipes later in this book)

Limit sodium intake. Sodium is abundant in processed foods (i.e. junk foods, chips, soda, etc.) so it's important to minimize your intake of those. Another good tip is to make sure that you read food labels properly. Choose products that say "low-sodium" or "sodium-free". It's important to make sure that you do not take more than 500 mg of sodium in a day.

Look for sugar-free food. Bloating is also caused by taking too much alcohol and sugar-laden food, so make sure that you don't take more than 2 to 3 servings of sugary food per day.

Eat 5 to 6 small meals instead of 2 to 3 big meals. Doing so will prevent you from feeling bloated, and will make it easy for your body to digest and metabolize what you have eaten. Plus, when you eat small meals, you get to keep yourself from feeling hungry over and over again.

Chew gassy vegetables and beans slowly. Potato, sweet potato, yam, cauliflower, broccoli, and other cruciferous vegetables can make you gassy—so take your time in chewing them. By eating beans regularly, your body will get immune to the gassy feeling—just make sure that you add small amounts only.

Try probiotics. Probiotics are simply good bacteria that keep the immune system healthy, and prevent bloating by regulating the digestive process. They also regulate the amount of good bacteria in the body.

Different Teas for Different Health Issues

Teas That Can Help With Fat Blocking

Not all teas are created equal. In this chapter, you will learn about teas that are known as fat-blockers—those that help break down fat, turn them into energy, and reverse fat storage effects, too!

What are those teas? Read on and find out!

Green Tea

Of course, it all starts with green tea!

This type of tea is so popular that in fact, it is already known as a post-workout staple. The thing about green tea is that its anti-oxidant properties easily break down fat that quickly boosts energy and hastens the metabolic rate. This way, even if you're not overly active, you can be sure that fat will still be burned—and that you will lose weight in no time!

Green tea also rehydrates the body and generally improves immunity!

Japanese Matcha Tea

Learning about the tea ceremony isn't just about appreciating art. It is also about knowing that Japanese tea is actually helpful in the sense that it increases thermogenesis (the use of heat to break fat down, and turn it into energy). From 8 to 10%, thermogenesis reaches a high of 35 to 48%! It lowers the amount of bad cholesterol, leaving you healthy and protected from heart diseases.

Pu-erh (Fermented Green Tea)

This type of tea is the kind that's fermented and then rolled into blocks. It helps lower levels of triglyceride compounds. Triglycerides are basically the dangerous kind of fat found in one's blood.

Aside from that, Pu-erh also lowers the amount of abdominal fat, even in high-fat diets—which is definitely a good thing!

Rooibos

The best thing about Rooibos tea is that it inhibits fat cell formation. You see, when there are no fat cells, there's also a very low chance that you will store lots of fat in the first place. By drinking Rooibos tea, you get to prevent fat cell formation by up to 22%!

Aside from that, Rooibos also prevents stress thanks to its unique combination of flavonoids. This way, your hunger is also suppressed—which leads to fat-burning, as well.

Barberry

Meanwhile, there's a kind of tea called Barberry—which is amazing because it prevents fat cells from growing bigger.

Barberry is made from the Barberry Shrub that is naturally known to prevent weight gain, even when one is on a high-fat diet.

More so, Barberry helps prevent the onset of insulin resistance, so it is safe to say that it is beneficial for diabetics, too. Barberry can also increase your energy levels. When your energy levels are high, you can do a lot of physical activities in a short amount of time. Likewise, when you're active, you prevent fat from taking over your body; and that's definitely a good thing!

Black Tea

While Barberry prevents fat cells from growing larger, black tea is responsible for reducing fat storage hormones in the body by decreasing cortisol levels. Cortisol is responsible for bad cholesterol and fat formation, and when it is shut down, it will be easier for your body to lose fat in your body.

It is best to drink black tea when you are stressed because it is during this time that adrenaline is able to break fat down, and release fat into your system to turn it into energy.

When Adrenaline and Cortisol work together, the body is able to break more fat down—and in turn, prevent the body from consuming more calories, too!

White Tea

White tea is the type of tea that's naturally sun-dried, which makes it full of anti-oxidants. The compounds found in white tea are able to block the formation of fat cells, as well as breaking fat down, and turning it into energy instead.

The antioxidant content, meanwhile, is able to trigger fat release from the cells and helps the liver turn the fat into energy, which, of course, is good for the body!

Incorporate these teas into your diet, and you will be able to start detoxing in no time.

Teas That Can Help With Metabolism Issues

Now, it's time for you to learn the type of teas that boost metabolism more than any other kinds of teas!

Porangaba Tea

Porangaba mostly grows in Brazil and other regions of South America, and is known as Brazil's very own weight loss potion. The leaves of the Porangaba plant resemble coffee. In fact, they also contain caffeine, but the amount is within the acceptable levels, and is not expected to bring forth undesirable side effects.

Porangaba acts as a diuretic that reduces appetite and naturally boosts weight loss. While it suppresses appetite, you can be sure that it will not damage your organs, making it a safe bet for weight loss!

It's best to drink a tea bag of Porangaba at least 30 minutes before each meal.

Star Anise Tea

Star Anise is native to China and has always been known to treat most digestive troubles, especially diarrhea and stomach upset.

Steep a whole pod in hot water for about 10 minutes to get the optimum effects of the tea. Make sure to strain and sweeten because drinking it without any other ingredient may make it too bitter for your taste.

Yerba Mate

Yerba mate is responsible for stimulating good cholesterol levels, and has long been known as the type of tea that can help prevent cancer.

What's great about yerba mate is that it has high anti-oxidant contents, which means that it is also rich in polyphenols and it hastens the activity of enzymes that break bad cholesterol down, and promote good cholesterol, instead.

It has been said that it is best to steep the tea in a squash gourd, and a metal straw must be used to drink it, too. You can also use a coffee maker to make the tea in; just put the pod where you usually put coffee grounds.

Peppermint Tea

The amazing thing about peppermint tea is the fact that it allows your body to control the amount that it eats. Peppermint tea actually speeds up digestion, which means that the metabolic rate will be higher, too.

You have to use the leaves of the peppermint plant to make your tea. Remember to add fresh or dried leaves to boiling water, and allow 4 to 5 minutes of steeping. Add some honey, if you want to. Take the tea hot or cold—it's up to you.

Oolong Tea

Oolong is a semi-fermented tea that burns fat up to 157% more than any other tea does.

Oolong is known to enhance metabolism, and is also used to prevent the body from absorbing more fat than necessary, which makes it an essential part of any weight loss diet program. Fat oxidation is blocked by up to 50% in just two weeks, and the tea can also be beneficial for those who suffer from heart ailments, and diabetes. It also prevents toothaches, and helps make the skin radiant, too.

The best thing about Oolong, however, is that it increases the level of plasma adiponectin in the body that is known to promote faster weight loss.

You can make oolong tea in just five minutes, more or less, if you want to. Just steep it in a cup of hot water. But for best results, steep it for 15 to 30 minutes.

Feiyan Tea

Feiyan Tea is mainly a combination of medicinal plants that can reduce the amount of fat that's accumulated by the body, and boost metabolic rate, especially when taken regularly. This won't be hard to do because this tea is known for having no chemical additives, and is also best consumed on a daily basis because it poses no side effect threats. By doing so, you can lose 5 to 8 lbs in just a month—or even less!

What's good about Feiyan tea is that it detoxifies the body, suppresses appetite, and also gets rid of extra, dangerous fat that your body doesn't need.

To make the tea, just soak a bag for around 5 to 10 minutes in hot water. You can start off by drinking the tea during your first night of the diet—so your body will have a better chance to adjust to it.

Rose Tea

And of course, there is rose tea, which is best known to prevent and treat constipation.

This tea is made from rose buds and flowers, and is known to be extremely therapeutic. It contains vitamins A, C, B3, D, and E that can help boost one's metabolism, prevent constipation, and also protects the body against infections.

To prepare the tea, make sure that you first clean the petals with the help of boiling water, then add 2 to 3 cups of the petals into a saucepan and boil for around 5 minutes. Strain and pour before drinking.

Teas That Can Help With Inflammation & Bloating Issues

Next, here are some teas that can help prevent bloating—and decrease inflammation at the same time.

White Lavender

This is basically a mix of white tea and French lavender. It has this light and somewhat romantic aroma, and is best for improving the intestine's mobility. This is possible because white lavender is able to stimulate gastric juice production.

Aside from bloat prevention, this tea is able to treat flatulence, colic, stomach pain, and indigestion.

Tulsi Honey Chamomile

This tea is abundant in antioxidants, and is also relaxing and soothing. It protects the digestive system and cleans the colon, thanks to the fact that Tulsi is actually considered as *Queen of the Herbs*, and has a high fiber content that helps detoxify the body.

It is also quite easy to drink as it kind of tastes like apple, but is definitely cooler and can help one feel and be in the moment. It keeps the nervous system healthy, as well.

Licorice

This sweet drink prevents constipation and keeps the body hydrated, thanks to its glycyrrhizin content.

Coconut Cocoa

This tea contains carob that has nutrients that keep the body safe from most diseases. It also has a naturally sweet and cooling flavor. It is perfect as a dessert, and can be added to other recipes, as well.

Tea Shanti

This Ayurvedic tea contains organic spearmint, orange peel, fennel, and basil. It is said that it can balance physical and spiritual elements in the body, which in turn can help the person become healthier. It also has loads of anti-viral and anti-bacterial properties. It keeps the immune system healthy, as well.

Ginger Tea

This keeps the body light and prevents bloating, even after eating a heavy meal! It invigorates your adrenals and also stimulates bowel elimination—which means constipation is easily prevented, and you will be able to look and feel healthy, too.

Peppermint Tea

Peppermint also prevents the body from bloating as it prevents gas and Irritable Bowel Syndrome. It strengthens stomach muscles, as well, which means fat-buildup will be avoided, too.

Fennel Tea

It is best to drink fennel tea after eating as it is a good digestive aid. This means that it hastens the metabolic process. Food will be easily digested and turned into energy, so your body can also get rid of fat quickly.

Fennel tea also prevents heartburn, gastrointestinal cramps, diarrhea, indigestion, and colic.

Teas That Can Help With Stress

Here are some teas that will help combat stress.

Valerian

Valerian may be a bit too strong for your taste, but it's still part of most detox diets because of the fact that it has amazing calming properties.

It works in two ways. One, it keeps you rejuvenated, and it also promotes better sleep habits. As they say, when you get enough sleep, it will be easier for you to do what you have to do. Valerian is actually recommended for people suffering from insomnia, and other sleep-related problems.

Passiflora Incarnate

This tea reduces headaches that have been brought on by stress and anxiety. When this happens, you get to release tension away from your body, so you will also be less irritated.

Also, it is great for women suffering from PMS and menstrual cramps, because it alleviates stress, and also lessens irritation that women usually suffer from during these times.

Linden

Linden is responsible for relaxing nerves and muscles, which of course, prevents stress and calms the mind.

Linden Tea is also recommended for people who often suffer from nerve tension, as well as stress-induced headaches. If you are no stranger to these, try to get yourself some servings of this tea.

Catnip

Yes, you can also try catnip!

Catnip prevents palpitations, and keeps you in an enthusiastic and excited demeanor. What's great about catnip is that it prevents digestion-related headaches. Sometimes, bloating and low metabolism happens when people suffer from the said condition—and that's why it's great to add catnip to your daily diet!

Lemon Verbana

This is another tea that is perfect for those with insomnia. It also combats nausea that is often brought on by an upset stomach.

Lavender

Tension headaches can be lessened with the help of lavender tea.

Lavender easily relieves stress, and can also help one sleep better, so it is advisable to have it as part of your regular diet if you have a sleep disorder. Lavender also works against anxiety and nervous exhaustion. It also regulates the digestive process; so with its help, you can be holistically healthy.

Skullcap

It is said that no other tea can help muscles relax any better than skullcap can. It reduces headaches, calms the nerves, reduces muscle spasms, and prevents muscle tension.

Also, women with PMS and menstrual cramps can benefit a lot from this tea. It alleviates pain and prevents further irritation.

Ginseng

Ginseng immediately clears out stress and mental exhaustion. Just after drinking a cup, you will already feel lighter, and you will feel at peace—which is extremely good, given the kind of life that most people live these days.

Ginseng can also help you sleep better, so do drink a cup during bed time.

Chamomile

Chamomile reduces indigestion and nausea, and can also calm the mind and soothe the soul; that's why it is often referred to as the tea that can drive stress away.

Hyperactive people also benefit from chamomile because it can easily stabilize one's mood, and it's perfect for those who suffer from insomnia,

Mint

Of course, with its amazing cooling properties, you can expect that mint is definitely part of this list. It relaxes the mind, and also prevents digestive upset—you really get to enjoy a lot of benefits with just one cup!

Foods to Eat

Here's a complete guide as to what you can and can't eat while on the flat belly diet—plus a diet plan for an entire week.

What You Should Be Eating

Nuts and Seeds. These must be eaten in moderation, and you should only go for those with low fat and calorie content (i.e., *linseeds, sunflower seeds, pumpkin seeds, chia seeds, almonds, and walnuts*)

Grains and Legumes. You definitely should eat a lot of these, but make sure you don't limit your meals to them in a day—make sure you add fruits and vegetables in the plan, too. Start with *whole meal pasta, brown rice, oats, quinoa, millet, red rice, and rye sourdough.*

Fruits and Berries. It's always best to stay organic as much as possible. *Pears, apples, lime, lemon, and grapefruit* are known for their detoxifying purposes—so please add them to your diet. Berries are also full of vitamins and antioxidants, which as you may know is an important part of the diet. Do eat *strawberries, raspberries, noni berries, goji berries, cranberries, blueberries, blackberries, and cherries. Watermelon* is also a good choice because it contains arginine—a chemical that boosts weight loss. *Bananas* also boost metabolism by up to 15%, as well. *Apples*, meanwhile, make sure you don't consume too much calories by burning fat enzymes away! They energize you a whole lot, too!

Vegetables. At least 9 vegetable servings per day, and make sure that they're mostly steamed or raw. Try *green leaf lettuce, arugula, collards, kale, turnip, leeks, radish, onion, cauliflower, Brussels Sprouts, mustard, and broccoli*, among others.

Chick Peas. Chick peas are great because they contain 2 grams of starch that block calories away.

Kidney Beans. Kidney beans contain lots of fiber and protein that your body needs to cleanse well.

Black Beans. Black beans are also amazing sources of protein, so add them to your diet.

Quinoa. Quinoa contains more than 8 grams of fiber and protein per serving, which makes it an amazing rice replacement.

Kale. Kale is the *King of All Greens*! It contains a lot of fiber and just 34 calories. It has calcium and iron, too.

Pears. By adding pears to your daily diet, you get 15% or more of your recommended dietary fiber per day.

Edamame. Edamame is also loaded with fiber and proteins, and is a good thing to munch on!

Dark Chocolate. At least ¼ serving of dark chocolate daily can give you a good amount of healthy fat, and can also block dangerous fat from entering the body.

Air-Popped Popcorn. There is a good reason Madonna and all these other celebrities swear by the popcorn diet. Three cups only have 100 calories, and have a great amount of fiber to keep you healthy, too.

Greek Yogurt. Greek yogurt contains calcium and protein that you need in your daily diet. It also is a great pro-biotic.

Eggs. Eggs should only be eaten in the morning. They are loaded with protein, and can help you get energized throughout the day.

Salmon. Salmon has the highest amount of Omega-3 fatty acids that naturally boost the body's metabolic rate, and can also prevent arthritis, heart ailments, and depression. It's the best lean meat you can eat.

Avocados. Of course, you also need fat in your system, but only the healthy kind. Avocados are surefire fruits that can give you the necessary healthy fat the body needs.

Oats. Oats, as well as cornflakes, are full of fiber that detoxify your system and can get you energized throughout the day.

What Else Can You Drink?

Now, here's a list of what you can drink while on the diet:

Tea. Herbal teas, as you may know by now, are an important part of your diet. Make sure you do not add sugar or milk, though. 3 to 5 cups per day is already good.

Water. Try to drink at least 1 to 2.5 liters per day. Make infused water (you can find recipes later in this book) to enhance flavor and not make drinking water a bit more "exciting" for you

Juice. Not the processed kind, though. Try to make your own green juices (with vegetables as base), and mix and match ingredients. It is actually fun, and can also help yourself gain a lot of nutrients by doing so. Try using the following: *cucumber, celery, beet, carrot, ginger, parsley, spinach, and cabbage.* Then add any of the following: *berries, watermelon, aloe vera, goji berry, acai berry, etc.*

Coconut Water. Coconut water is dubbed as nature's own sports drink that has a thermogenic effect, and helps make sure that the gut is strong and safe.

Shakes and Smoothies. Shakes and smoothies are fine, as long as you make them yourself, and they do not contain additives.

What Might Be Your Downfall
And of course, here is a list of foods that you have to avoid while on the diet:

Saturated Fats. These include: *larm, palm oil, coconut oil, cheese, butter, whole wheat dairy products, chicken with the skin, and high fat meat (i.e., pork, lamb, and beef)*

Trans Fats. These include: *candy bars, fried foods, vegetable shortening, stick margarine, packaged snacks, baked pastries (i.e., pizza, cakes, doughnuts, cookies)*

Dairy Products. *Cheese, milk, butter.*

Table Salt

Sugar

Artificial Sweeteners

Flavored Drinks. *Cordial, Soft Drinks, etc.*

Alcoholic Beverages. *Beer and spirits, wines, etc.*

And What to Eat Instead

As you can't use the mentioned food products above, here's what can you use instead.

Salt. Try to use sea salt, or herbal seasonings (i.e., liquid aminos)

Dairy. You can use butter/margarine, organic milk, oat milk, soy milk, almond milk. You can also use yogurt, which is also proven to be one of the healthiest snacks around.

Dressings. Use apple cider vinegar, lemon juice, or cold pressed olive oil. Liquid aminos and stevia, instead of honey, are good, too.

Sugar. Try maple, brown rice, bran syrup, and raw honey.

The First Seven Days

Here's a sample meal plan that you can follow to help you get started on the diet!

Day 1
Breakfast: Berry Bowl (made with slivered almonds, coconut yogurt, and a mix of berries)

Lunch: Farro and Summer Peas plus Watermelon Salad

Dinner: Roast Salmon and Lemon Chickpea Burgers

Snacks: Strawberries with unsweetened yogurt

Teas to drink: Green, Roobois, Lavender

Day 2
Breakfast: Quinoa and Sweet Potato Fritters with Wilted Spinach

Lunch: Vegetable Stir Fry with Kelp Noodles

Dinner: Zucchini Noodles with basil and tomatoes

Snacks: 1 apple and 10 raw almonds

Teas to drink: Green, Japanese Matcha, Chamomile Tea, Barberry

Day 3
Breakfast: Cinnamon and Honey Spiced Grapefruit

Lunch: Baked Cauliflower Florets with cumin powder and sweet paprika

Dinner: Roasted Tomato Soup

Snacks: a handful of raw nuts

Teas to drink: Star Anise, Yerba Mate, Rose, Green Tea

Day 4:

Breakfast: Scrambled eggs with flat-leaf parsley and chives with smoked trout

Lunch: Spicy Balsamic Avocado Salad and 100grams grilled prawns

Dinner: Vegetable and Lentil Soup

Snacks: Cucumber Sticks with 2 Tbsp Hummus

Teas to drink: Roobois, Green, Peppermint, Rose, Porangaba

Day 5:

Breakfast: Quinoa Porridge with slivered almonds, cinnamon, strawberries, blueberries, grated apple, and almond milk

Lunch: Grilled Chicken Salad (made with asparagus spears, sliced red onions, cherry tomatoes, and mixed lettuce)

Dinner: Tina Nicoise with Salsa Verde

Snacks: fresh grapefruit and 5 walnut halves

Teas to drink: Green, Oolong, Chai, Yerba Mate, Barberry

Day 6:

Breakfast: Hemp protein shake with unsweetened almond milk, frozen blueberries, and chia seeds

Lunch: Zucchini and Egg Muffins

Dinner: Steamed Snapper with Quinoa Tabbouleh

Snacks: Carrot Sticks with Peanut Butter

Teas to Drink: White Lavender, Feiyan, Black Tea, Oolong, Japanese Matcha

Day 7:

Breakfast: Poached Egg with Mushrooms and Grilled Spinach

Lunch: Corn and Roasted Sweet Potato Salad

Dinner: Spinach Salad with Roasted Pumpkin, toasted walnut, and spiced apples

Snacks: cucumber sticks with hummus

Teas to Drink: Rose, Black Tea, Green Tea, White Tea, Peppermint

Get Moving

You also have to make sure that you complement your diet regimen with the proper exercises that will help you lose weight, and keep your health in check. Here's what you can do:

First Week

Yoga

Light Weights

30 Minute Walk

Rest (on Thursday)

Bikram Yoga

Pilates and Yoga

60 Minute Walk/Hike

Second Week

Body Weight Exercises

Rest (on Tuesday)

Swim

Yoga

45 minute walk

Rest (on Saturday)

Bikram Yoga

Don't Forget the Superfoods

Superfoods are foods that contain a lot of nutrients—that really makes them, well, super!

In other words, these foods are those that can boost the immune system, and make the tea cleanse work better—and of course, that's important when you want to make sure that your immune system is healthy, and that tea cleanse will work well for you.

Here's what you need:

Coconut Oil. As mentioned in an earlier chapter, you also need to exercise so that your body adjusts to the diet. Coconut oil can help you with that because it converts fat into energy by hastening metabolic rate. Of course, when you have more energy, it will be easier for you to exercise in a regular manner, and you will be able to follow your plans, as well. Add a tablespoon of this superfood to your breakfast smoothie and you're all set!

Also try: *Coconut Oil Waffles, Coconut-Curry Lentil Stew, Coconut Curry Pumpkin Soup, Coconut Lime Rice, Coconut Walnut Squash*

Chia Seeds. Oh, Chia Seeds. They became popular recently because of the fact that they contain many antioxidants and multivitamins that make them a great part of any diet. Chia seeds also increase brain function because of their high Omega-3 fatty acid content. They also prevent heart diseases and stroke by bringing bad cholesterol levels down. Chia seeds also contain calcium, iron, minerals, vitamins, amino acids, fiber, and proteins that the body needs to grow properly. They're mildly sweet, and you can eat them on their own, or together with other ingredients in a smoothie.

Also try: *Chia Lemon Loaf, Chia Shake, Chia Seed Pudding, Chia Brown Rice and Egg, Chia Breakfast Pudding, Chia Seed Mousse*

Goji Berries. Goji Berries have long been popular in Japan and some Asian countries for their natural healing strength. They contain more than 20 vitamins and minerals, and are said to help balance hormones, fight viruses, and strengthen eyesight. They also boost longevity of life—by making sure that your body is well-adjusted to the change; and that your brain can adjust to it well, too. Add around ½ cup of goji berries to your breakfast smoothie and you're all set; it will definitely perk you up.

Also try: *Goji Juice, Goji Trail Mix, Goji Jam, Goji Balls, Goji Relish*

Flax Seeds. Flax Seeds have high fiber and fatty acid content. They also soften the skin and make it radiant, while strengthening the joints, and keeping brain and immune system healthy. Toxins can also be eliminated from the body with the help of flax seeds. They have a nutty flavor and can also be easily added to your healthy smoothies!

Also try: *Flax Seed Porridge, Flax Seed Soup, Flax Seed Chutney, Flax Seed Cookies, Flax seed Sandwich*

Acai. Acai is a Brazilian berry that contains fiber and protein, and easily energizes the body. Many weightlifters add acai in their diet because it strengthens their bodies, as well as their immune system, and it also tastes good—A bit like chocolate. Add a tablespoon of this superfood in your smoothie and you're good to go!

Also try: *Acai Superfood Bowl, Acai Puree*

Camu Powder. Camu is rich in Vitamin C. It keeps you safe from viruses and also strengthens your immune system in the process. Camu also keeps the skin vibrant and healthy, and can be eaten with any fruit. Its flavor blends with fruits well. Add a tablespoon or so to your smoothies in the morning.

Also try: *Camu Pasta Dough, Camu Tenderizer, Camu Energy Bars, Camu Vegan Ice Cream*

Hemp Protein. As the name suggests, this superfood is full of protein and is best eaten during childhood because it helps children grow well, and can also repair and strengthen muscles. Again, it's perfect for gym buffs and weightlifters. If hemp protein isn't available, you can buy hemp hearts and add it to smoothies or salads to give them a nutty kick!

Also try: *Hemp brownies, hemp cereal, hemp porridge, hemp muffins*

Avocado. Avocado contains more than 20 vitamins and minerals that boost the immune system and can keep you satiated for a long time.

Also try: *Avocado Guacamole, Grilled Chicken salad with Avocado, Avocado, Lettuce, and Tomato Sandwich*

Cacao Powder and Nibs. Cacao keeps you safe from colds and flu, and is also filled with antioxidants that keep your skin glowing and healthy. Two to four tablespoons of cacao powder mixed with breakfast smoothie is enough to energize you throughout the day.

Also try: *Cacao energy bars, cacao protein shake, Vegan chocolate mousse*

Spirulina. Spirulina is probably the worst-tasting superfood — just based on its algae-like taste — but it is super high in nutrients. It has a lot of omega acids and protein. To mask the taste, just add a teaspoon to your breakfast smoothie and you won't even notice it's there.

Also try: *Fried Tofu with Spirulina, Spirulina Nut Butter Bites, Spirulina Ice Cream with Lychees*

14 Quick & Easy Fat Busting Smoothies!

In this chapter, you will learn about tea smoothies that you can prepare in just around 90 seconds—that can really help you lose weight! Check them out below.

Peaches and Green Tea Smoothie

This is a great detoxifier, and will definitely help you lose weight while building your muscles up, too! This smoothie is something that most gym buffs swear by!

Ingredients:

½ peach

1 cup brewed Green Tea

1 scoop Vanilla Soy-Protein Powder

Instructions:

Mix all ingredients together in a food processor or blender, and process until smooth. It is a good idea to drink green tea shortly before drinking this blend so your body can be prepared for it.

Green Tea and Chai Smoothie

With the heat coming from Chai spice, and caffeine from green tea, you can be sure that fat will be burned, and your metabolism will be hastened—all thanks to this smoothie!

Ingredients:

A pinch of cardamom

A pinch of cinnamon

½ inch ginger root

1 serving Vanilla Chai

1 cup ice

1 banana, peeled

1 cup green tea, chilled

Instructions:

Using a high-powered blender, mix all of the ingredients together and process until smooth.

Serve and enjoy!

Matcha Banana Smoothie

If you need something that will wake you up and make sure you do not consume a lot of calories throughout the day, try this Matcha Banana Smoothie! It's like drinking coffee—minus the side effects!

Ingredients:

½ cup ice

1 serving French vanilla yogurt

1 cup non-dairy alternative

1 tsp Matcha green tea powder

½ frozen banana

Instructions:

Mix all of the ingredients in a blender and process until smooth.

Serve and enjoy!

Creamy Lavender Earl Grey Smoothie

This one could be your instant pick me up if you need an afternoon snack that will not make you put on the pounds. This is something that you absolutely have to go for!

Ingredients:

½ tsp Himalayan rock salt

½ tsp lavender buds

1 tsp cinnamon

1 serving French vanilla yogurt

1 tbsp. hemp hearts

1 cup cold Earl Grey Tea

½ cup light coconut milk

6 Earl Grey Tea ice cubes

Instructions:

First, make the Earl Grey Tea in boiling water.

After making the tea, set it aside for it to cool down.

Pour the tea in ice cube trays and put in the freezer.

Then, mix all of the ingredients together in a food processor or blender and pulse until smooth.

Serve topped with coconut ribbons, if desired.

Chamomile Tea Smoothie

Chamomile has this calming and relaxing effect that's sure to keep the stress away. Historically, chamomile has also been used to prevent and treat digestive disturbances, and is also best taken after a stressful or strenuous activity to refresh your mind and body!

Ingredients:

1 serving natural yogurt

¼ cup ice

1 tsp lemon juice

½ tsp fresh grated ginger

½ cup frozen peaches

1 cup chilled chamomile tea (brewed for at least 5 minutes)

Instructions:

For at least five minutes, make sure to steep chamomile tea and keep it chilled.

Then, mix ingredients with chilled tea in a food processor or blender. Pulse until smooth, and serve.

Enjoy!

Rooibos Tea Smoothie
This smoothie is one of the best you'll ever taste. It's decadent and rich, and could definitely wake you up—even when you're extremely tired!

Ingredients:

½ serving protein vanilla powder

1 tsp coconut oil

2 tbsp. hemp seeds

1 vanilla bean pod, scraped

1 ½ cups warm Roobois tea

Instructions:

Keep the tea warm first, and then add it to the hemp hearts, coconut oil, and vanilla bean in the blender, and pulse on high speed until creamy.

Then, add protein powder and blend for 30 seconds more.

Serve and enjoy!

Cayenne Chai Matcha Smoothie
Spice up your day and burn more fat with this amazing blend!

Ingredients:

Ice

¼ tsp cayenne powder

½ inch fresh ginger

1 ½ cups coconut milk

1 serving vanilla chai powder

½ frozen banana

Instructions:

Mix all of the ingredients in a blender or food processor.

Serve and enjoy!

Yerba Mate Smoothie

It's said that this tea-smoothie has Peruvian roots, and has been used even in ancient times as an energizer!

Ingredients:

2 ice cubes

1 tsp maca powder

1 tbsp. cashew butter

1 frozen banana

1 serving French vanilla powder

1 cup Yerba Mate tea, unsweetened

1 ½ cups unsweetened milk alternative

Instructions:

First, make a cup of Yerba Mate tea and then set it aside to let it cool.

Then, mix all of the ingredients in a blender, together with Yerba Mate, and process until smooth.

Serve and enjoy!

Almond and Sweet Potato Surprise

This recipe will balance electrolytes and fluids in your body, and also give you more protein, too.

Ingredients:

½ sweet potato

A handful of almonds (soaked in water at least for a few hours or overnight)

½ orange

1 apple

Instructions:

Combine all the ingredients in a juicer, and pulse until smooth.

Serve and enjoy! You can add ice if desired.

Beet Carrot Ginger Mix

With only 155 calories, you can be sure that this recipe won't make you pack on the pounds in any way!

Ingredients:

½ apple

½ beet

1 carrot

A few slices of ginger

Instructions:

Combine all the ingredients in a juicer or blender, and pulse until smooth.

Serve and enjoy!

Super Green Smoothie

With Kale, also known as the *King of all Greens* as its main ingredient, you can be sure that this is one of the healthiest drinks you can try!

Ingredients:

A bunch of kale leaves

Cucumber

Green grapes

Granny Smith Apple

Instructions:

Mix all of the ingredients in a blender or food processor and pulse until smooth.

Serve cold and enjoy!

Cherry Pear Mix

This smoothie contains only 192 calories, and is also full of antioxidants that will surely help you look and feel better!

Ingredients:

½ glass of cherries

1 apple

1 pear

Instructions:

Combine all of the ingredients in a juicer and blend until smooth.

Serve and enjoy!

All the Berries

Berries contain many antioxidants that can help make your skin beautiful and supple, and can also boost enzymes that aid in weight loss! Check it out.

Ingredients:

3 or 4 middle sized strawberries

A glass of blueberries

1 mango

Instructions:

Combine all the ingredients in a blender or juicer.

Serve and enjoy!

Orange and Kiwi Surprise

Kiwi is high in Vitamin C—which means that healing processes will be easier, and that your immune system will generally be stronger, too!

Ingredients:

A pinch of cinnamon

Oranges

Grapefruit

Kiwis

Instructions:

Combine all of the ingredients in a juicer, and pulse until smooth.

Serve and enjoy!

Stay Hydrated. 14 Fat Busting Water Infused Drink

Grapefruit and Lemon-Infused Water

With the help of this recipe, toxins in your digestive tract will be lessened, and your body can release more water.

Ingredients:

½ lime, sliced

½ lemon, sliced

2 to 3 mint leaves

½ cucumber, sliced

½ grapefruit, sliced

½ gallon spring water

Instructions:

Mix all of the ingredients together in a pitcher and chill for at least 2 hours before serving.

Enjoy!

Cinnamon and Apple Detox Water

The blend of ingredients used in this recipe has been proven to boost one's metabolism—and it's easy to make, too!

Ingredients:

1 cinnamon stick

1 thinly sliced apple

Instructions:

First, make sure that the apple slices are on the bottom of the pitcher.

Add the cinnamon stick and pour water in.

Chill for around 10 minutes and then serve and enjoy!

Strawberry and Kiwi Detox Water

This recipe will kick free radicals away—which means that your colon will be clean, and your body will be safe from toxins! This has amazing anti-inflammatory properties as well!

Ingredients:

Ginger

10 to 12 Mint leaves

1 medium sized sliced cucumber

1 sliced lemon

2L water

Instructions:

Combine all of the ingredients in a pitcher and let steep in the fridge overnight.

Serve and enjoy!

Mint and Watermelon Combo

This recipe is perfect for the summer due to its amazing cooling properties!

Ingredients:

2 to 3 mint leaves

½ cubed watermelon

2L water

Instructions:

Combine all of the ingredients in a pitcher and let steep in the fridge overnight.

Serve and enjoy!

Rosemary and Strawberry Vitamin Water

This drink is extremely hydrating and also contains a good amount of antioxidants.

Ingredients:

Filtered water

A dash of coarse salt

2 sprigs fresh rosemary

2 cups watermelon, cubed

1 cup strawberries

Instructions:

In a bowl, mash strawberries and rosemary together.

Then, add the ingredients in a pitcher with watermelon before pouring water inside.

Keep in the fridge for at least 4 to 6 hours.

Serve and enjoy!

Fruity Cucumber Energizing Water

This one is known to be totally refreshing, and can also prevent digestive troubles.

Ingredients:

Fresh mint

Sliced pears

Sliced cucumbers

Peeled grapefruit

Raspberries

A pitcher of spring water

Instructions:

Mix all of the ingredients in a pitcher and refrigerate for at least 2 hours.

Make sure to drink throughout the day!

Lemon Cucumber Surprise

Here's another refreshing drink that has amazing anti-inflammatory properties and is also full of antioxidants that will help keep you in shape.

Ingredients:

10 mint leaves

1 lemon, sliced or wedged

1 cucumber, sliced or wedged

8 cups water

Instructions:

In a pitcher, mix all the ingredients together and let it steep overnight before serving.

Enjoy!

Cinnamon and Apple Cider Refresher

While it may not be for the faint of heart, this one definitely has all the healing and antioxidant properties that you need. It clears the digestive tract, too.

Ingredients:

½ sliced apple

½ tsp stevia raw sweetener

1 tsp cinnamon

1 tbsp. fresh lemon juice

1 to 2 tbsp. apple cider vinegar

12 oz. water

Instructions:

Mix all of the ingredients (with the exception of apples) in a blender and process for around 10 seconds.

Add apple slices.

Serve and enjoy!

Ginger and Lemon Detox Water

This is a powerful drink because it drives toxins away from the colon, and also strengthens the digestive tract. It heightens the metabolic rate in the process, too.

Ingredients:

½ inch ginger root knob

½ lemon juice

1 12 oz glass water, room temperature

Instructions:

Grate ginger using a zester, and add lemon juice to the glass of water.

Serve and enjoy!

Aloe Water

Aloe is not only good for the hair; it's good for the body. It detoxifies the digestive tract, and helps your skin glow!

Ingredients:

A pitcher of water

Lemon juice

Aloe Vera

Instructions:

Wash and rinse aloe vera.

Split the leaf in half and then scrape the gel and place it in a container.

Then, mix gel with lemon juice and water.

Keep in the fridge for at least 30 minutes and then serve and enjoy!

Orange and Blackberry Detox Water

The combination of blackberries and orange means that you will be able to drink something that has amazing anti-inflammatory benefits, and is full of antioxidants, too.

Ingredients:

Ice

A handful of blackberries

2 Mandarin oranges cut into wedges

6 cups water

Instructions:

Mix all of the ingredients in a pitcher and keep chilled overnight before serving.

To intensify the flavors more, you can squeeze orange juice into the blackberries first.

Enjoy!

Watermelon Detox Water

Watermelon is already a good hydrant in itself. When mixed with water, it gives you this ultimately refreshed feeling that can help you get through a long day.

Ingredients:

4 cups water

2 cups seedless watermelon, cubed

Instructions:

Put watermelon in pitcher and cover with water.

Let the recipe sit for a few hours before serving.

Enjoy!

Sugarcane Pineapple Surprise

This has just the right amount of acidity that will help balance PH in your body—and keep you safe from diseases too!

Ingredients:

Ice

4 to 5 large pineapple chunks

2 sticks sugar cane

2L purified water

Instructions:

Mix all the ingredients in the pitcher, and stir.

Let it sit as long as you want so the water gets infused with nutrients even more.

Mint Raspberry Detox Water
This one is best consumed during lunch—especially on hot summer days!

Ingredients:

1 lime

2 tbsp. fresh mint leaves

2 tbsp. fresh or frozen raspberries

2L cold spring water

Instructions:

Microwave lime for at least 30 seconds to get more flavor, and then slice before adding to the mint and raspberries in a jug.

Pour water in the jug and chill for at least 2 hours before serving. Enjoy!

Common Ailments That Tea Can Help Heal!

(Again, always consult your doctor before taking the advice of this, or any other publication)

Here is a guide on the various diseases the Flat Belly Tea Diet can cure or prevent for you.

Heart Diseases

Studies show that green tea lowers LDL or bad cholesterol by up to 35%. When this happens, the heart will be protected and strokes can be prevented.

More so, tea can also prevent fat buildup. Usually, heavier people are more susceptible to heart diseases because fat is already abundant in their bloodstream. When tea is part of one's regular diet, the more it protects the body from elements that may damage the heart.

One Japanese case study has shown that 4 out of 5 men who have added tea to their diet have shown life longevity—without any heart problems!

Cancer Prevention

Research has it that with the help of catechins, a form of antioxidant found in tea, free radicals are sought and destroyed on the spot. When free radicals are destroyed, the body is spared from most life-threatening diseases including cancer.

A study done in *McGill University* shows that tea's antioxidants are able to shrink tumors that are mostly found in mice. Lung cancer risk is also lessened by up to 18%, also due to tea.

Now, when one has already suffered from cancer in the past, relapse can be prevented with the help of tea in the sense that an increase of green tea intake prevents cancer cells from forming, mostly by destroying mitochondria, which are responsible for creating cancer cells in the body.

Pancreatic, colorectal, and prostate cancer are prevented, as well.

Liver Health

Consuming tea is also good for the health of your liver. Remember, liver produces bile, which is an important part of the digestive tract that regulates digestive processes. When the liver is healthy, the whole body is healthy, too.

With the help of catechins found in tea, redness of the liver is prevented. You see, when someone's liver is red, there's a chance that it is unhealthy. Green Tea can aid in making sure that the liver stays healthy.

Tea also cleanses the after-effects of alcohol, making sure that even after alcohol intake, the liver doesn't get damaged—but make sure you don't consume too much alcohol. Whatever people eat may also build toxins in the liver—so it's important for it to be kept clean at all times.

With the help of tea, toxin and ammonia buildup in the liver can be prevented.

Arthritis Support

Arthritis happens because of inflammation. If you've been reading this book properly, you'll know that there are actually various kinds of tea that help prevent inflammation, especially when combined with other ingredients.

Compounds found in tea reverse the effects of responses that are usually associated with arthritis, diabetes, and other inflammatory problems.

The breakdown of cartilage walls is also prevented, making sure that arthritis patients are safe from further damage. Tea helps keep a person's condition stable, instead of letting it worsen—and that's one of the best things that tea can do.

Normalizes Blood Sugar Levels

Another amazing thing about tea is that it can help normalize blood sugar levels, and doing so will help prevent the onset of one of the most debilitating diseases out there—Diabetes.

This happens because tea regulates the body's glucose levels, and turns glucose to energy. Now, when this happens, the body will be stronger, and will be able to use the energy for more important things, instead of letting a disease consume the body.

It's a Great Digestive Aid

Thermogenesis—the term given to "fat to energy" conversion—is increased by at least 8 to 10 % when someone uses tea in his daily diet. This not only burns fat, but also regulates the digestive process.

Tea also reduces intestinal gas, and can also prevent certain diseases from happening, such as ulcers, ulcerative colitis, and Chron's Disease.

More so, weight grain is prevented because tea is able to suppress one's appetite, without making the body prone to ulcer and gastro-enteritis. It doesn't only prevent weight gain; it reduces one's weight, too.

While losing weight, fat is oxidized and turned into energy—and this is done at the same time blood cholesterol levels are being lowered. This is mainly caused by polyphenols found in tea—they promote healthy and fast metabolism.

Antioxidant Booster

As said earlier, tea is full of antioxidants that slow the process of aging down, and that also wards of disease. Tea also repairs damaged cells and makes sure that free radicals do not get to them. More so, these antioxidants prevent the growth of cancer cells, keep cholesterol under manageable levels, and dilate blood vessels to improve energy and elasticity in the body. This also prevents clogging of the blood, and makes sure there's proper antioxidant concentration in the body.

Strengthens the Neurons

When neurological processes are restored and protected, you'd get to protect yourself from Alzheimer's Disease and memory loss. Degenerative diseases are also prevented.

This happens because tea contains L-Theanine, an amino acid that promotes better neurological health—and not a lot of food products are able to do this!

Prevents Dehydration

Unlike coffee and soda, tea keeps the body hydrated, and makes sure that dehydration is prevented. Tea has moisture, as mentioned in an earlier chapter, which means that it actually has water, unlike flavored or carbonated drinks.

And, it's a Great Immune Booster

As often reiterated in this book, you can expect that with the help of tea, the aging process is slowed down—so you can still look and stay healthy even while you're growing older. Studies done have shown a lot of promise when it comes to tea's effects on the immune system.

Remember, tea is something that you can add in your daily diet. Don't try to let all the myths about it fool you. It's definitely amazing and safe!

You Have Questions?

Q: What makes the Flat Tea Belly Diet healthy? What are the nutrients that one can get from tea?

A: As there are various kinds of teas, you can expect that nutritional content varies, too. But mostly, you can expect that you'll get the following:

Moisture. Moisture is basically tea's water content—and everyone knows how important water is to one's daily life. Tea moisture helps stabilize the processes done by organs of the body, which means that you will be holistically healthy in the long run. Some people don't like to drink water too much, so the fact that they get to drink various kinds of tea means they'll still get to fill their body's need of water.

Lipids. Lipids are good kinds of fat that are mostly mixed with protein and can help hair become stronger.

Protein. Protein is one of the most important nutrients that the body needs to function well. You can get at least 2% or more from one cup of tea.

Carbohydrates. Tea contains around 4 to 5% carbohydrates, so you can omit rice and other grains from your diet.

Calcium and Phosphorous. These are both needed for bones to grow strong. Your teeth can benefit from these nutrients, too.

Potassium. Potassium helps cells do their job properly. Tea contains a lot of potassium.

Fluorine. Fluorine helps make teeth stronger.

Magnesium. Magnesium is essential for the strength and growth of the human body, and can also help prevent tissue breakage.

Sodium. Sodium prevents hypertension.

Also, you can expect that by regularly drinking tea, you will get to fill your dietary needs by getting:

6% Vitamin B6

25% Vitamin B2

9% Vitamin B1

10% Zinc

16% Calcium

Around 50% of flavonoids and anti-oxidants

Q: Caffeine isn't good for the body, and tea also contains caffeine, right?

A: The latest studies show that moderate amounts of caffeine can in fact aid the body, especially in weight loss.

However, tea contains less caffeine than coffee does, and the amount that it contains has been proven not to be detrimental to one's health. Even though some brands of tea contain a lot of caffeine, it is usually much less than found in coffee grounds.

Also, keep in mind that tea's caffeine content is based on the parts that have been used for certain recipes—so one really cannot generalize. Mostly, you can expect caffeine content based on the particular part of the plant such as:

Lower stem – 1.40% caffeine

Upper stem – 2.40% caffeine

Third Leaf – 2.90% caffeine

Second Leaf – 3.50% caffeine

First Leaf – 4.20% caffeine

Bud – 4.70% caffeine

Q: But how much caffeine should one take daily?

A: According to the *American Official Food Guide*, one must only consume around 400 to 450 mg of coffee each day (3 to 5 cups) which when calculated is equivalent to around 10 to 12 cups of tea.

In short, you won't exceed the recommended caffeine content just by drinking tea. However, you have to make sure that you do not drink coffee while drinking tea. When you're on a tea diet, a single cup of coffee can give you around 200 milligrams of caffeine already—and that's a lot, considering you have a lot more tea to consume. In short, self-discipline is important.

Q: It's said that green tea contains a lot of antioxidants. What are antioxidants and how much is contained in green tea?

A: Antioxidants are basically healthy chemicals that protect the cells from free radicals, which are harmful for the cells because they pose the threat of cell damage. When free radicals are thwarted, you won't easily age, and you will still look radiant over time. Antioxidants also prevent heart diseases and stroke from happening.

Speaking of green tea, it's often said that it contains the most number of antioxidants as compared to other teas. However, research and recent studies show that black tea is also capable of doing what green tea does. Black tea, in particular, reduces the risk of cancer as it easily targets cells that can cause cancer in time.

Basically, you can expect that you'll get these from tea:

Gallocatechin – 3 to 4%

Catechin – 1 to 2%

Epigalllocatechin Gallate – 9 to 13%

Epigallocatechin – 3 to 6%

Epicatechin – 1 to 3%

Q: So, does this mean that tea is good for healthy aging?

A: Yes, absolutely.

Since tea restores the skin's elasticity due to its antioxidant content, healthy aging is promoted. Take for example those in countries that naturally drink tea (i.e., Japan)—you can see that they age gracefully, compared to those who just drink tea occasionally, and whose diets are mostly made up of preservatives.

Research also has it that those who drink tea live longer—without having to worry about diseases that old age brings.

Q: Can tea also prevent Alzheimer's Disease?

A: According to a number of studies done over the years, especially those performed by the *University of Newcastle*, tea actually improves memory, and when one's memory is good, Alzheimer's can be prevented in the long run.

This is because tea affects the cholinergic system of the brain, which, when damaged, contributes to the risk of getting Alzheimer's in the future. Tea hydrolyses the enzymes that destroy the said system, and therefore gets to protect the brain from further damage.

Also, studies have shown that tea contains the same elements as pharmaceutical products do—minus the side effects, and while working for a long period of time. This means that the effects will not only be prevalent today, but as long as one has tea in his diet.

Q: Is tea bad for pregnant women?

A: First and foremost, this is just a myth.

Studies show that drinking tea has no effects to either the pregnant and lactating mother, or to her child, whether through growth retention, or miscarriages. There are also no effects of tea caffeine on child development and mental processes.

However, when one already has an aversion to tea, and often suffers from indigestion when consuming caffeine, it's best to consult the doctor first before drinking tea. It's also best to eat a healthy diet and exercise regularly even when one is pregnant, so that giving birth will be easy, and so the woman will be able to maintain good health while taking care of her child, as well.

A pregnant woman may drink up to 3 to 4 cups of tea each day, but has to refrain from coffee as it may bring forth palpitations.

Q: What about decaffeinated tea? Is it good, too?

A: Decaffeinated tea is made through solvent-based extraction. While caffeine is taken away from coffee, you can expect the nutrients to stay intact, so yes, it's actually good for your health.

Q: Can tea prevent stroke?

A: When taken regularly, yes.

This is because tea contains polyphenols and antioxidants that the body easily absorbs to protect itself from free radicals that may lead to stroke and cancer. While doing so, tea also clears the digestive tract, and can also protect one from most degenerative diseases.

Q: What is real tea?

A: As the name suggests, real tea is basically just tea in its original form—or derived naturally, such as by drying, leaf maceration, withering, and the like. Tea that can be bought bottled in the grocery store isn't real tea.

Mostly, real tea, especially when talking about green tea, is one that comes from the Camila Sinensis plant. This plant makes tea suitable as a beverage, and it's always best to get hold of it, rather than buy tea from the market. You can get more nutrients from real tea than processed tea, that's for sure.

Q: Can overcooked water affect the quality of tea?

A: Yes, it can.

You know, tea actually tastes better when polyphenols and caffeine meet each other, and work together—and this only happens when you get to brew tea properly, and not in overcooked or over boiled water.

Overcooked water dampens the taste of the tea. When it's no longer palatable, you may feel like you shouldn't add it in your diet anymore—and that's what you have to prevent it from happening.

Q: Will I have to urinate all the time because I'm on a tea diet?

A: Not really. Compared to coffee, tea won't make you urinate that much.

Q: It's said that tea blocks iron absorption. Is this true?

A: Absolutely not.

Dietary iron has two forms, which are non-heme iron (plant iron), and heme iron (animal iron). When you drink tea, your body still gets to absorb at least 15 to 35% of heme, and 25% of non-heme iron—which means you'll get the amazing dietary benefits that they bring.

It is also easy to absorb polyphenols and ascorbic acid with the help of tea.

Q: And, is tea really good for my immune system?

A: Yes, especially when you take it regularly. This is because it boosts the body's capability to bring infection down, and it also tracks germs better—so the immune system can drive them away from the body.

In short, if you want to live a healthy life, you definitely must include tea in your diet!

Conclusion

I hope that with the help of this book, you now realize the great benefits of tea, and why it's important to add it to your diet.

I hope that you're willing to try the recipes mentioned here, and the various kinds of teas for different occasions.

Who knows? You might just become a tea ceremony master, too!

For now, remember it's important to take care of your health and drinking tea can help you along this journey

Finally, if you enjoyed this book, please take time to post a review on Amazon. It will be greatly appreciated.

Melinda

About the Author

Melinda is an Amazon Best Selling Author, cooking and freezing expert, loomer, crocheter, and mom of three. Melinda has been preparing healthy, delicious and inexpensive home cooked meals for her family for the past several years. She is also an avid tea drinker but confesses to sometimes sneaking in a morning coffee.

As a "Thank You" for downloading this book, Melinda would like to offer you a FREE copy of one of her other books" The Raw Deal. The Real Benefits of Eating Raw for Health and Weight Loss. To get your free copy, just visit her website melindarolf.com

Melinda lives with her husband, 3 children 2 dogs, a cat, and a yellow bellied turtle in Swanville, Maine

Other Books in the "Home Life" Series by Melinda Rolf

101 DIY Household Hacks

The Wheat Belly Lifestyle

Prep Freeze Serve

Prep Freeze Serve Chicken

African Black Soap & How to Make It

How to Make Natural Handmade Soap

Loom Jewelry for Beginners

The Superfood Power Smoothie Book

Crockpot Recipes

Halloween

Meatless Eating

MELT Your Pain Away

The Raw Deal: Raw Food Lifestyle

Inside Crochet

Clean Eating

Planning the Perfect Christmas

Paleo Christmas

Paleo Thanksgiving

Mason Jar Recipes.

Mason Jar Gifts

Available at Amazon and other fine stores in e-book and paperback format

Printed in Great Britain
by Amazon